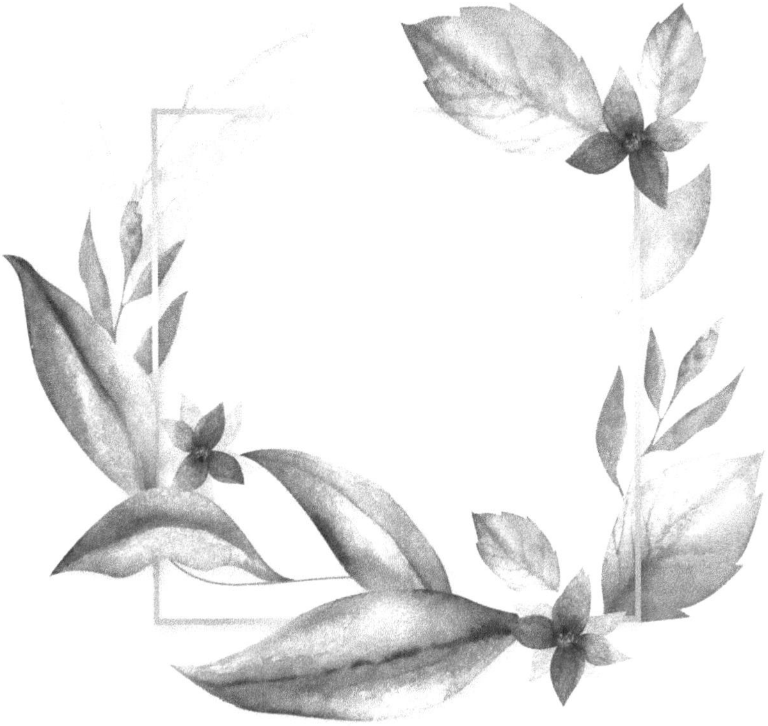

This Notebook Belongs To

www.ingramcontent.com/pod-product-compliance
Lightning Source LLC
Chambersburg PA
CBHW070420220526
45466CB00004B/1482
* 9 7 8 1 6 5 9 9 3 5 4 3 1 *